# THE SYPHILIS SELF-TEST

## A Complete Guide to Understanding, Accessing, And Using At-Home Testing.

Lorinda Innis

**Table of Contents**

# Chapter 1

## *The Unexpected Comeback of Syphilis*

The history of syphilis in the United States is replete with amazing highs and lows, spanning many centuries and shedding light on human behavior, society, and medicine. Few illnesses in the history of public health have undergone such a drastic transformation as syphilis. It was once a scourge that plagued decades, and after almost disappearing from the American scene, it has made a startling and unexpected reappearance in recent years.

We must first consider the near-eradication of syphilis in the late 20th century in order to fully understand the importance of its reappearance. With the discovery of penicillin in the 1940s, medical practitioners at last have a potent weapon against this archaic adversary. The effect was immediate and significant. As syphilis rates fell, public health experts began to envision its complete eradication by the 1990s. In 2000, the National Plan to Eliminate Syphilis was introduced by the Centers for Disease Control and Prevention (CDC), an audacious endeavor that seemed capable of accomplishing its lofty objective.

The hope was not misplaced. The most contagious phases of the illness, primary and secondary syphilis, had decreased to only 2.1 instances per 100,000 persons by 2000, the lowest level since records started in 1941. Decades of focused work that combined extensive antibiotic usage, effective public health initiatives, and raised awareness and education led to this incredible accomplishment.

Nevertheless, the festivities were fleeting. Syphilis was quietly making a return, even as health experts were planning methods for the last push towards eradication. The early 2000s saw a little but steady rise in the number of instances recorded, which signaled the beginning of problems. These increases were first mostly limited to certain groups, especially men who had sex with men (MSM). However, as time went on, it became harder to ignore the pattern.

From its low point in 2013, the incidence of primary and secondary syphilis has more than quadrupled to 5.3 cases per 100,000 individuals. Even more concerning was the fact that the increases were now occurring in a variety of demographic categories rather than just one or two. The grim reality of an epidemic that was on the rise had taken the place of the fading ideal of eradication.

This unanticipated turnaround has many intricate and varied causes. Dating apps contributed to changes in sexual behavior, such as a decline in the usage of condoms and an increase in the number of partners. The issue was ironically exacerbated by the success of HIV medications, as fewer people were concerned about safe sex practices and AIDS-related anxiety subsided. Many public health services were left unable to handle the growing danger as a result of financial cuts. The opioid crisis and the syphilis revival also coincided because drug use was linked to a more risk-taking attitude and less access to healthcare.

By the time we get to the present, things have only become worse. The CDC's most current statistics presents a dismal picture of syphilis in the US. The number of syphilis cases recorded in 2022 exceeded 207,000, which is a record since the 1950s. Compared to 2018, this is a startling 80% growth in only four years.

There is no one group or area that is excluded from the surge. Although the number of males who have sex with men remains disproportionately high, rises have been seen across all age categories, genders, and locations. The increase in congenital syphilis infections, or situations when the infection is transferred from mother to child during pregnancy or delivery, is especially concerning. The last 10 years have seen a more than tenfold rise in these instances, a heartbreaking reversal of progress that underscores the larger shortcomings in combating the disease.

There is an actual public health emergency in the United States over syphilis. It puts a burden on the healthcare system, has an impact on the community, and presents serious difficulties for people and families. The disease's dramatic reappearance serves as a sobering reminder that improvements in public health are never certain and need ongoing attention and work to sustain.

Understanding syphilis itself is crucial to appreciating the seriousness of this situation. This includes knowledge of the disease's biology, mode of transmission, and its consequences if left untreated. Treponema pallidum, a tiny, spiral-shaped bacteria that has afflicted humans for generations, is the cause of syphilis. It is an especially sneaky enemy because of its multi-stage development and ability to imitate other illnesses.

There are four phases that the illness usually develops through, each with unique dangers and symptoms. At the location where the bacteria entered the body, a single sore known as a chancre often appears to signal the start of the main stage. This sore may go undetected and is generally painless, particularly if it is in an area that is difficult to see. The infection advances to the secondary stage if therapy is not received, although the chance will cure on its own in three to six weeks.

A variety of symptoms, such as fever, enlarged lymph nodes, muscular pains, and skin rashes, are indicative of secondary syphilis. These might be sporadic symptoms that last for weeks or months. Again, if treatment is not received, the illness progresses to a latent stage in which no outward symptoms of infection are present. Years or even decades may pass during this dormant phase.

Tertiary syphilis is the last and most severe stage of the disease. At this stage, the infection has the potential to harm the heart, brain, and neurological system, among other organ systems. It may result in mental disease, blindness, deafness, or even death. Despite the fact that tertiary syphilis is less common now that medicines are readily available, it's possible repercussions highlight the need for early identification and treatment.

Sexual intercourse with an infected individual, including vaginal, anal, and oral sex, is the main way that syphilis is spread. Tiny cracks in the skin or mucous membranes allow the germs to enter the body. Syphilis may be transmitted from pregnant mothers to their fetuses, which can result in serious health issues or even fetal death.

The effects of untreated syphilis go much beyond the patient. Because syphilis sores make it simpler for HIV to enter the body, they aid in the transmission of the virus. Significant pregnancy difficulties, such as stillbirth and infant mortality, may result from it. With millions of dollars being spent on complications management and treatment, there is a significant financial burden.

Furthermore, those who are impacted by the social stigma attached to STDs may have severe psychological effects. People may be discouraged from seeking testing and treatment out of fear of prejudice or judgment, which will further accelerate the epidemic's growth.

The present syphilis outbreak in the US is a complicated social problem in addition to a medical one. It touches on themes of socioeconomic inequality, healthcare access, education, and cultural perspectives on sexual health. It needs a multipronged strategy that goes beyond treating individual patients to combat this recurrence.

The fact that syphilis is often asymptomatic, particularly in its early stages, is one of the main obstacles in treating disease. Many syphilis patients are unaware that they have the illness, which permits it to worsen and perhaps spread to other individuals. This emphasizes how crucial routine testing is, especially for individuals who are more vulnerable.

It is recommended by the CDC that all expectant mothers have a syphilis test at their first prenatal appointment. At least once a year, males who have sex with other men, those living with HIV, and those who have several sexual partners should be tested. These suggestions, however, won't do much unless individuals can easily obtain healthcare and feel at ease doing so.

The syphilis pandemic is significantly influenced by healthcare inequities. Rural locations and low-income urban districts are among the communities that often experience a disproportionate share of the disease's impact. Any plan for reducing syphilis that is successful must address these differences.

Another essential element in the battle against syphilis is education. Many individuals, particularly those in younger generations, may not be aware of the symptoms and indicators of syphilis or might not think it poses a serious risk. It is crucial to provide comprehensive sex education that includes information on syphilis and other STDs.

Concerns over the future of syphilis therapy have been raised by the emergence of antibiotic-resistant bacterial strains. There have been instances of resistance to various antibiotics used to treat syphilis, despite the fact that penicillin is still quite successful in treating the illness. This emphasizes the need of continued investigation and monitoring to guarantee the sustainability of available treatment solutions.

The infrastructure of public health is essential to the management of syphilis and other STDs. One of the most important methods for stopping the spread of syphilis is contact tracing, which involves finding and alerting an affected person's sexual partners. Unfortunately, a lot of public health agencies lack the tools necessary to complete this time-consuming procedure successfully.

The issue is made more complicated by the convergence of the syphilis epidemic with other public health emergencies, such the opioid crisis and the current COVID-19 pandemic. These related issues put a burden on healthcare resources and may cause funds and attention to be diverted from efforts to prevent syphilis.

Technology presents possibilities as well as obstacles in the fight against the recurrence of syphilis. Social media and dating apps have been linked to encouraging dangerous sexual conduct, but they also open up new channels for outreach and education. These platforms have been tested by certain health departments as a means of sharing information on testing and prevention.

The development of quick, point-of-care syphilis testing has the potential to greatly increase the number of cases diagnosed and treated. These tests may provide answers in a matter of minutes, enabling the start of therapy right away. It is still difficult to guarantee that these tests are widely accessible and used.

The first over-the-counter, at-home syphilis test was just approved by the FDA, which might be a major breakthrough in the battle against the illness. With only a drop of blood, anyone may use this NOWDiagnostics test to screen for syphilis in the comfort of their own homes. This invention may help remove some of the obstacles to testing, especially for those who may be hesitant to seek treatment because of stigma or lack of access, even while it is not a substitute for expert medical care.

There are no simple answers as we struggle with the sudden resurgence of syphilis. The recurrence of the illness is a complicated subject that speaks to larger problems with our healthcare system and society at large. It will need consistent work, creative thinking, and a readiness to face up to hard realities about sexual behavior and health to address it.

The American syphilis narrative is far from finished. What may be accomplished with coordinated public health measures is shown by its near-elimination in the late 20th century. Its return is a sobering reminder of the need for ongoing awareness. The lessons we take away from this unanticipated return will be critical in determining how we address syphilis and other public health issues going ahead.

Eliminating syphilis is just one aspect of the battle against it; another is building a culture in which all people have access to the knowledge, tools, and support they need to preserve their sexual health. It's all about dispelling the stigma and encouraging candid, open discussions about sexual health. It's about treating public health concerns holistically and acknowledging their interdependence.

We need to maintain our optimism while we face the difficulties brought on by the syphilis recurrence. The human resourcefulness and perseverance that previously almost completely eradicated syphilis might be used once again. We can stop this epidemic and move toward a day when syphilis is no longer a growing danger but rather an uncommon occurrence with redoubled dedication, enhanced tactics, and continuous research.

# Chapter 2

## *The Alarming Trends*

Over the last ten years, there has been a sharp increase in syphilis infections in the United States; the alarming increase occurred between 2018 and 2024. Public health authorities are not the only ones who are concerned about this growth; medical professionals and the general public are also concerned. The data presents a startling image of an illness that was almost eradicated in the United States but has now made a startling comeback.

The Centers for Disease Control and Prevention (CDC) estimated that 115,000 cases of syphilis in all stages were recorded in 2018. The number of cases increased dramatically to over 207,000 by 2022, a rise of 80% in only four years. Final figures are still being gathered, but early data indicates that this trend will continue until 2023 and 2024. The rate of increase has far surpassed the expansion in the population, suggesting that there has been a true increase in the frequency of illness rather than just better techniques for reporting or detection.

Further dissecting the data exposes even more alarming trends. Particularly notable increases were seen in primary and secondary syphilis, the two most contagious phases of the illness. About 35,000 cases of primary and secondary syphilis were recorded in 2018. This figure increased by 71% to over 60,000 cases by 2022. The sharp rise in syphilis cases overall may be partially attributed to this spike in the disease's most contagious phases, because more people in these stages resulted in greater rates of transmission.

Throughout this time, there has been a change in the regional distribution of syphilis cases. Sexually transmitted illnesses (STIs), including syphilis, have traditionally been more common in urban regions, but between 2018 and 2024, there was a noticeable shift in STI prevalence toward suburban and rural locations. States with historically low syphilis rates started to report notable rises. For instance, by 2022, some Midwestern states with less than 200 cases in 2018 were reporting more than 500 cases. The absence of infrastructure and resources in many rural regions has hindered public health responses to this geographic extension of STI epidemics.

The statistical analysis's disproportionate effect on certain demographic groupings is among its most startling findings. Men who are sexually involved with other men (MSM) remain one of the most impacted groups. Approximately 54% of all cases of primary and secondary syphilis in 2018 belonged to this group. Even while the rate had somewhat dropped to around 45% by 2022, the overall spike in cases meant that the total number of cases in this demographic had climbed dramatically.

But there were also concerning rises in syphilis incidence among heterosexual men and women between 2018 and 2024. Specifically, the percentage of cases among women increased throughout this period at a quicker pace than that of cases among males. About 14% of instances of primary and secondary syphilis in 2018 were in women. This has risen to about 20% by 2022. There are important ramifications to this change, particularly with relation to the possibility of congenital syphilis.

Notable trends have also been seen in age demographics. All age groups are susceptible to syphilis, but the 25–34 age range has consistently recorded the largest number of cases. Nonetheless, there were alarming rises in both younger and older age groups between 2018 and 2024. Between 2018 and 2022, cases for those aged 15 to 24 climbed by almost 65%, while cases for people aged 45 and beyond grew by roughly 50%. These patterns imply that in order to successfully target a larger variety of age groups, public health messages and actions must be customized.

Throughout this time, syphilis rates have continued to differ by race and ethnicity and have even become worse in some circumstances. The populations of African Americans and Hispanics continue to be disproportionately impacted. 5.6 times as many African Americans as non-Hispanic Whites had primary and secondary syphilis in 2018. This difference has widened by 2022, with rates among African Americans being 6.2 times greater than those among non-Hispanic Whites. Though to a little lesser extent, Hispanic populations saw similar tendencies.

Particularly concerning increases have also been seen in Native American and Alaska Native populations. Between 2018 and 2022, the incidence of syphilis cases surged by over 200% in certain states with sizable Native populations. The aforementioned gaps underscore the persistent influence of social determinants of health, such as healthcare accessibility, socioeconomic position, and institutional inequities in public health education and outreach.

One of the most concerning developments of this era is the sharp rise in congenital syphilis cases, which may be directly attributed to the rise in syphilis cases among women of reproductive age. Congenital syphilis is the result of a syphilis-affected pregnant mother infecting her fetus. Serious repercussions may ensue, including as stillbirth, neonatal mortality, and chronic health issues for the surviving babies.

In the United States, 1,306 instances of congenital syphilis were documented in 2018. This figure increased to 3,761 instances by 2022, a startling 188% rise in only four years. This upward tendency seems to have persisted in preliminary data for 2023 and 2024, while final figures are still being produced. Congenital syphilis is typically avoidable with appropriate prenatal care and prompt treatment of infected mothers, thus this increase in incidence is very concerning.

Congenital syphilis has increased, although not everywhere in the nation. Compared to other states, some have witnessed even more extreme increases. For instance, between 2018 and 2022, Texas recorded a 384% rise in congenital syphilis cases, whereas California had a 232% increase in the same time frame. These regional disparities in public health responses, prenatal care usage, and healthcare access are indicative of variances throughout the nation.

The differences seen in adult syphilis cases are reflected in the demography of congenital syphilis cases. Newborns who identify as African American or Hispanic experience rates that are many times greater than those of non-Hispanic white newborns, indicating a disproportionate impact. Congenital syphilis was more common in African American newborns (8.3 times higher) and Hispanic infants (3.5 times higher) in 2022 compared to non-Hispanic white infants.

Gaps in prenatal treatment have also been brought to light by the rise of congenital syphilis. Mothers who get inadequate or no prenatal treatment account for a considerable fraction of occurrences of congenital syphilis. About 40% of congenital syphilis infections in 2022 were linked to moms who had just had treatment in the third trimester or had not received any prenatal therapy at all. This emphasizes how crucial timely and reliable prenatal treatment is to avoiding congenital syphilis.

There are grave repercussions from the increase in congenital syphilis. Syphilis-related stillbirths and newborn mortality more than quadrupled between 2018 and 2022. There were more than 220 documented stillbirths and infant deaths from syphilis in 2022 alone. For babies who survive, there may be serious long-term health effects, such as developmental delays, convulsions, blindness, and deafness.

The rise in instances of congenital and adult syphilis has put a burden on public health resources and brought attention to flaws in the American healthcare system.

Numerous municipal and state health agencies have found it difficult to keep up with the increasing number of cases, especially in regions where syphilis rates had previously been low. Budgets and staff have been overworked because of the need for contact tracing, testing, and treatment, often taking resources away from other crucial public health programs.

The COVID-19 pandemic added to the complexity of public health measures during this syphilis outbreak. During the peak of the epidemic, several STI clinics temporarily shuttered or scaled down operations, which restricted access to testing and care. Disruptions in the supply chain also resulted in shortages of drugs and testing supplies, such as Benzathine penicillin G, the recommended treatment for syphilis.

There have been suggestions for a greater emphasis on syphilis prevention and control as a result of the trends shown between 2018 and 2024. Increased financing for STI prevention initiatives, greater access to testing and treatment, and focused outreach to the most impacted groups are all priorities, according to public health authorities. Additionally, there has been a drive for improved STI screening integration into standard medical treatment, especially for women who are pregnant or who are at greater risk.

The emergence of syphilis around this time has also brought attention to how interrelated many public health issues are. For example, the opioid crisis has been connected to higher incidence of syphilis and other STIs because drug users may be more prone to swap drugs for sex or participate in high-risk sexual activities. This emphasizes the need of all-encompassing strategies that deal with many public health concerns at once.

A sobering reminder that the fight against infectious illnesses is not always linear is provided by the concerning patterns in syphilis incidence between 2018 and 2024. A disease that was once almost completely eradicated in the US has returned and is now a serious public health concern that affects a variety of people all throughout the nation. The necessity for focused treatments and the persistence of health inequalities are highlighted by the disproportionate effect on certain demographic groups.

It is especially alarming that the number of instances of congenital syphilis has skyrocketed, indicating that some of society's most defenseless citizens have not been adequately protected. Congenital syphilis is a preventable disease, and every occurrence highlights how vital it is that pregnant women get prompt treatment and have access to prenatal care.

Lessons from this era of syphilis comeback must guide future public health initiatives as we go ahead. Reversing these alarming trends will need continued financing for STI prevention initiatives, more awareness, and better access to testing and treatment. In addition, long-term success against syphilis and other STIs will depend on tackling the underlying social and economic causes of health inequalities.

Syphilis cases from 2018 to 2024 are statistically analyzed to provide a clear picture of a serious public health concern. It emphasizes the need of ongoing watchfulness, creative methods of treatment and prevention, and a dedication to tackling the many variables that lead to the spread of STDs. We can only expect to put syphilis rates back under control and safeguard the health of present and future generations by persistent work and a comprehensive strategy.

# **Chapter 3**

## *Barriers to Detection and Treatment*

The recent syphilis revival has highlighted a number of barriers that prevent this dangerous STD from being detected and treated effectively. These obstacles need to be carefully examined and specifically addressed since they are complex and have their roots in social, economic, and cultural issues.

An important obstacle in the battle against syphilis is the widespread stigma attached to STIs (sexually transmitted illnesses) in general. Many times, this stigma makes people reluctant to seek medical help, even when they think they may have been exposed to or developed syphilis. Many individuals choose not to be tested for STIs or seek treatment because of the immense shame and humiliation surrounding them.

The occurrence of this stigma is not new. STIs are medical illnesses, but historically, they have been seen as a sign of moral failure or promiscuity. Even with improvements in medical knowledge and care, many cultures still hold these harmful and antiquated beliefs. A major barrier to getting treatment is the fear of being judged by partners, friends, family, or medical professionals.

Furthermore, the stigma associated with syphilis and other STIs may have an impact that goes far beyond one's own health. If someone's status is discovered, it may cause interpersonal tension, social isolation, and potentially affect job and housing chances. Particularly in cases when a patient is asymptomatic or exhibiting only moderate symptoms, the apparent advantages of being tested and treated are often outweighed by the dread of these social and economic consequences.

Healthcare professionals are essential in maintaining or eradicating this stigma. Some patients claim that when they seek STI testing or treatment, medical staff members make them feel guilty or ashamed. These unfavorable experiences may deter people from seeing the doctor for follow-up treatment or in the future if they have health issues. Conversely, medical professionals who treat STI patients with professionalism, empathy, and a lack of judgment may assist in dismantling these barriers and promote more candid conversations about sexual health.

There are other reasons why people are reluctant to seek medical attention than simply stigma. Many people, especially young adults, might feel awkward or ashamed to talk to a healthcare professional about their sexual health. Cultural taboos around sex, unfamiliarity with the healthcare system, or the sensitive nature of the subject matter may all contribute to this unease. Because of this, even when they have concerns about their sexual health, many individuals may put off or avoid getting treatment.

Accessibility is a major obstacle to syphilis diagnosis and treatment, especially in underprivileged areas. These access problems might be of many different kinds, such as financial hardships, language and cultural limitations, or physical restrictions.

Access to medical institutions that provide STI testing and treatment might be restricted in many remote regions. People may have to travel great miles to go to a clinic or hospital, which may be difficult for people who don't have a dependable way to get about or can't take time off from work. Due to the geographical barrier, diagnosis and treatment may be delayed, which may enable the illness to worsen and perhaps spread to other people.

There are unique access challenges in urban settings. Even though there are more healthcare facilities, they are often overworked and understaffed, which leads to lengthy wait times for visits and outcomes. When local clinics cannot accommodate the demand for STI testing and treatment services, people may be forced to seek care elsewhere or postpone treatment.

One major factor restricting access to syphilis diagnosis and treatment is financial obstacles. The expense of STI testing and treatment may be unaffordable for those without health insurance or with high deductible plans. Copays and deductibles may be quite expensive, even for those with insurance, particularly for low-income individuals and families. Even when someone believes they may have been exposed to syphilis, many people may choose not to seek treatment out of concern of incurring large medical expenditures.

In addition, there is a dearth of medical professionals in many marginalized areas, especially those who specialize in sexual health. This scarcity may result in overburdened healthcare professionals, hurried scheduling, and inadequate treatment. Care obstacles may often be exacerbated by the necessity for patients to see many different doctors or schedule several sessions in order to get a diagnosis and treatment.

Accessibility problems in underprivileged areas are often exacerbated by language and cultural obstacles. It may be especially difficult for immigrant communities and non-English speaking people to navigate the healthcare system. Inadequate provision of culturally sensitive treatment and language interpretation services may result in misinterpretations, incorrect diagnoses, and a reluctance to seek further medical attention.

Furthermore, getting access to healthcare may be particularly difficult for members of several vulnerable communities, including drug users, sex workers, and the homeless. These populations often face prejudice and may decide not to seek medical attention out of concern for potential legal consequences or disapproval from medical professionals. Mobile clinics and outreach initiatives may aid in closing this gap, but more all-encompassing solutions are required to guarantee that all groups have fair access to syphilis diagnosis and treatment.

The general lack of knowledge and education on the illness is the third significant obstacle to efficient syphilis control. Even with the recent increase in instances, a large number of individuals are still unaware about the signs, causes, and treatments of syphilis. Delays in identification, greater transmission, and worse health consequences might result from this information gap.

The widespread dearth of thorough sexual education in many communities and schools is one of the main problems. Many people grow up without having a thorough grasp of sexually transmitted infections, such as syphilis. People may find it challenging to identify symptoms, comprehend their danger variables, or choose when to be tested and treated as a result of this fundamental ignorance.

Furthermore, it is simple to ignore or confuse the symptoms of syphilis with those of other illnesses. Many people mistakenly think they have recovered from syphilis without treatment since the first stage of the disease often manifests as a painless sore that heals on its own. Diagnosis might be made more difficult by the secondary stage's vast variety of symptoms that can resemble those of other disorders. Without the right information, people could not identify these symptoms as possible syphilis symptoms, delaying treatment and raising the risk of transmission.

There is more to the lack of awareness than just identifying symptoms. The major long-term effects of untreated syphilis, which include harm to the heart, brain, and other organs, are not well known to many individuals. A careless approach to diagnosis and treatment may result from this ignorance of the infection's possible seriousness.

Moreover, the mode of transmission of syphilis is often unclear. The majority of individuals are aware that it may be transferred via intercourse, but less are aware of the danger of transmission from actions like kissing or the potential for congenital syphilis to be transferred from mother to unborn child during pregnancy. This ignorance may result in unsafe actions and the loss of preventative possibilities.

Healthcare professionals are not exempt from the educational divide. Since syphilis rates have been low for a long time, some medical personnel may not be as knowledgeable about the symptoms and appropriate diagnostic techniques as they need to be. This may make it more difficult to stop the illness from spreading by resulting in missed diagnosis or ineffective treatment.

In order to remedy this lack of knowledge and instruction, public health programs are crucial. These initiatives, nevertheless, often encounter obstacles of their own. The scope and regularity of awareness efforts may be restricted by financial limitations. Furthermore, since STIs are sensitive, it may be challenging to spread knowledge in certain conservative areas or via conventional media outlets.

The emergence of digital platforms and social media poses obstacles as well as new avenues for awareness and education. These channels may be useful for reaching younger audiences, but they can also spread false information. It takes constant work and adjustment to new communication methods to make sure that the public is informed about syphilis in a trustworthy and accurate manner.

The ignorance about testing alternatives and methods is another facet of the education divide. A lot of individuals may not be aware of the testing procedure, where to be tested, or how often they should get examined. This problem is compounded by the new availability of at-home testing methods, which many people may not be aware of or may not trust.

Insufficient knowledge and instruction can play a role in the persistence of stigma. Myths and false information about syphilis and other STIs may promote unfavorable preconceptions and stifle candid conversations about sexual health. In order to break this pattern, it's important to provide a space where honest and judgment-free conversation about sexual health is encouraged in addition to offering accurate information.

To overcome these obstacles to syphilis diagnosis and treatment, a multimodal strategy is needed. Increasing education and awareness, expanding access to treatment, and lowering stigma must all be prioritized simultaneously. This might include creating focused outreach programs for marginalized populations, educating healthcare professionals in providing culturally competent and nonjudgmental treatment, and initiating extensive public health campaigns that make use of both conventional and digital media.

The involvement of policymakers is critical in removing these obstacles. This might include boosting financing for services related to sexual health, putting in place measures to safeguard patient privacy, and requiring thorough sexual education in schools. Furthermore, looking into cutting-edge solutions like mobile health clinics and telemedicine may be able to assist underprivileged populations in overcoming some of their access challenges.

In order to adequately handle the syphilis recurrence, the healthcare system itself must change. This can include incorporating STI screening into regular check-ups with medical professionals, enhancing communication between various healthcare providers and public health organizations, and using technology to expedite the testing and treatment procedures.

Advocacy groups and community organizations are also crucial players. These organizations may provide resources and information, support legislative changes that will enhance syphilis treatment and diagnosis, and act as a link between underprivileged communities and healthcare institutions.

One potentially game-changing development in removing some of these obstacles is the availability of at-home syphilis testing alternatives. For those who may be unwilling to be tested in a professional environment because of stigma or accessibility concerns, these tests might provide a discreet, practical choice. But for these tests to be effective in stopping the syphilis recurrence, they must be reliable, inexpensive, and used correctly.

In light of the unexpected resurgence of syphilis as a significant public health issue, removing these obstacles to diagnosis and treatment is imperative. We may attempt to stop this return and build a future in which syphilis is no longer a rising concern by addressing the problems of stigma, access, and education head-on.

# Chapter 4

## *The Game-Changer: At-Home Testing*

Innovation in the field of sexual health often presents both opportunities and difficulties. In the continuous fight against sexually transmitted infections (STIs), the U.S. Food and Drug Administration (FDA) has authorized NOWDiagnostics' First To Know Syphilis Test, which is momentous. The first at-home, over-the-counter syphilis test was introduced with this invention, which was disclosed on August 16, 2024. It has the potential to completely change the way people think about their sexual health.

The First To Know Syphilis Test from NOWDiagnostics is a revolutionary approach to STI screening. Syphilis testing has only been available in clinical settings for many years, requiring patients to contact medical professionals for blood samples and ensuing laboratory processing. This new test offers a degree of privacy and ease not before possible for syphilis detection, bringing the power of diagnosis right into people's homes.

One of the test's most notable aspects is how straightforward it is. The test just requires one drop of blood from the user, and results are ready in fifteen minutes. The anxious wait for findings is one of the main obstacles to STI testing, which is addressed by this quick turnaround time. The First To Know test has the potential to lessen some of the psychological difficulties related to STI screening since it offers almost instantaneous response.

The test, which costs $29.98, is designed to be affordable for a variety of customers. The fact that it is expected to become available in the second half of 2024 is significant since the incidence of syphilis in the US is rising at an alarming rate. The need for creative screening techniques has never been greater, with cases rising by 80% between 2018 and 2022 and total reported cases surpassing 207,000 in 2022 alone—the largest number since the 1950s.

The First To Know Syphilis Test procedure is intended to be as simple to use as possible. Users are advised to use an alcohol swab to wipe their fingers after opening the test kit. They puncture their finger with the supplied lancet to draw a little amount of blood. The diagnostic procedure is then started by applying this drop of blood on the test strip. The blood sample starts to flow over the strip when it comes into contact with the test's chemicals.

If syphilis-specific antibodies are present in the blood, they attach to antigens on the test strip throughout this period.

The test makes use of immunochromatographic technology, which has been simplified and made more portable for use at home. With the use of this technique, syphilis antibodies may be visually detected by looking for colorful lines on the test strip. Users may examine these lines to understand their findings after the 15-minute waiting time. For syphilis antibodies, one line denotes a negative result and two lines, a positive result.

Any diagnostic test must be reliable, but it's particularly important for home usage tests. The First To Know Syphilis Test properly detected positive specimens 93.4% of the time, according to clinical studies by NOWDiagnostics. For a screening test, this high sensitivity is essential because it reduces the possibility of false negative results, which can cause treatment to be postponed and the illness to spread further.

It's crucial to remember that the First To Know test is not perfect, just like any screening tool. The FDA and NOWDiagnostics strongly stress that positive findings should be followed up with confirmatory testing by a healthcare professional since false positives and false negatives may happen. This two-step method seeks to strike a compromise between diagnostic accuracy and accessibility by having a home screening followed by a professional confirmation.

Syphilis testing at home has several potential benefits that are not to be overlooked. The biggest advantage is probably that it's more accessible. The test reduces the entrance barrier for syphilis screening by doing away with the need for an initial doctor's visit. This is especially crucial for those who may be unwilling to be tested because of stigma, a lack of time, or difficult access to medical facilities.

Another important benefit is privacy. More individuals may be encouraged to screen for syphilis if they may do it in the privacy and comfort of their own home, particularly if they are uncomfortable discussing their sexual health in a professional environment. This greater openness to testing could result in early diagnosis and treatment, which might stop the virus from spreading.

It is impossible to exaggerate the convenience element. Without having to make appointments or travel to clinics, people may easily learn about their syphilis status with results accessible in as little as 15 minutes. The simplicity of use and quickness of this test might encourage more frequent testing, which would be in line with public health guidelines for STI screening at regular intervals among sexually active people.

Furthermore, underprivileged communities with limited access to healthcare services may be reached by the First To Know test. In rural areas, for example, lack of healthcare professionals and geographic constraints can make it difficult for residents to be tested for sexually transmitted infections. This gap might be filled by at-home testing, giving those who would not otherwise be tested access to an essential health service.

The development of at-home syphilis testing does, however, have some restrictions and possible negative effects that need to be properly taken into account. The possibility of incorrect findings interpretation is one of the main worries. Even while the test is meant to be simple to take, there's always a chance that people won't comprehend or interpret their findings correctly, which might cause them to feel unnecessarily anxious or reassured.

The test's incapacity to differentiate between illnesses from the past and present is another drawback. Since syphilis antibodies may linger in the blood for a long time even after treatment is effective, a positive First To Know test result does not always signal that an infection is still active. This emphasizes how crucial it is to get follow-up testing results and speak with medical professionals to decide if therapy is necessary.

There's also a chance that people may depend only on tests conducted at home and neglect to seek appropriate medical attention. Although the test instructions explicitly indicate that confirmatory testing is required in the event of a positive result, there is no assurance that users will take this action. This may result in lost chances for counseling and treatment, which might let the virus worsen or spread to other people.

Another factor to think about is the psychological effects of getting a good outcome at home without having quick access to expert advice and assistance. A favorable outcome may cause considerable anxiety for some people, which emphasizes the need for strong support networks and readily available, understandable information about options and future steps.

The possible consequences of widespread at-home syphilis testing are significant from the standpoint of public health. These tests have the potential to greatly increase the number of individuals who are aware of their syphilis status if they are widely utilized. In order to stop syphilis from spreading and from having more serious long-term health effects, such as harm to the heart, brain, nerves, eyes, and other organs, early identification is essential.

The population's overall prevalence of syphilis may decline as a result of the higher testing rates prompting more prompt treatment. Considering the recent increase in instances, including those involving babies, this is especially crucial. The number of cases of congenital syphilis, which happens when a woman transmits the virus to her unborn child while she is pregnant, has increased tenfold in the last 10 years. Pregnant women may benefit from at-home testing to detect and treat illnesses, which would stop the diseases from spreading to the unborn child.

Additionally, the pressure on healthcare systems may be somewhat reduced by the availability of at-home testing. Clinics and hospitals may be able to concentrate their resources on the confirmation, management, and treatment of positive cases if people are permitted to do early tests at home. This might increase the overall effectiveness of syphilis therapy.

Additionally, the First To Know Syphilis Test might be an effective instrument for focused public health initiatives. These tests might be given out by health departments during outreach programs or in neighborhoods at high risk, thereby reaching people who would not otherwise be tested. The disproportionate impact of syphilis on certain populations, such as males who have sex with men and certain racial and ethnic minority groups, may be addressed by this focused strategy.

The actual effects of at-home syphilis testing on public health, however, will rely on a number of variables, such as test uptake rates, test use guidelines, and follow-up advice compliance. Healthcare professionals and public health authorities will need to devise plans to guarantee that at-home testing enhances comprehensive STI prevention and treatment initiatives rather than taking their place.

In order to maximize the advantages of at-home syphilis testing while minimizing any possible disadvantages, education will be essential. Widespread distribution of easily understood instructions on how to conduct the test, evaluate findings, and seek follow-up treatment is required. Healthcare professionals should also be educated, since they will need to be ready to answer queries and concerns from patients who have taken at-home exams. This education should not stop with test takers.

The real-world effects of at-home syphilis testing will need more study and observation, as with any new medical technology. Research looking at how these tests impact the prevalence of syphilis overall, treatment start rates, and testing rates would be very helpful in developing future public health initiatives.

An important advancement in the battle against syphilis has been made with the approval of NOWDiagnostics' First To Know Syphilis Test. Testing in the house may raise screening rates, encourage early diagnosis and treatment, and ultimately lessen the toll that syphilis has on both people and society. Nevertheless, cautious execution, thorough training, and interaction with current healthcare systems are necessary for its success. As we go, realizing the full potential of this new tool in managing sexual health will depend on striking a balance between innovation and appropriate usage.

# **Chapter 5**

## *Moving Forward: Strategies and Solutions*

To combat the recurrence of syphilis, a multimodal strategy is needed. The use of at-home testing in comprehensive care techniques has been more effective. The First To Know Syphilis Test from NOWDiagnostics was approved by the FDA, which is a big step toward enabling people to take charge of their sexual health. This novel testing strategy removes a number of obstacles that have traditionally prevented syphilis diagnosis and treatment.

Traditional clinical facilities cannot match the privacy and convenience offered by at-home testing. The stigma around sexually transmitted diseases (STIs) may be a major barrier to testing for many people. This psychological barrier is removed by being able to take a test in the comfort of one's own home, which may lead to a higher test-taking rate. Additionally, the accessibility of these tests may encourage more frequent testing, which is essential for early diagnosis and intervention.

But it's important to understand that at-home testing is not a stand-alone fix. It needs to be seen as an additional instrument in a larger healthcare system. These tests are not conclusive diagnostic instruments, even if they provide a preliminary screening. For confirmation and treatment, positive findings from at-home testing need to be followed up with expert medical attention. This emphasizes how crucial it is to have open lines of communication and to educate people about the drawbacks of at-home testing as well as the essential next actions.

It is important to carefully assess how to include at-home testing into comprehensive treatment methods. It is imperative that public health authorities and healthcare practitioners provide precise instructions on how to integrate these tests into current processes. For those who test positive, this entails putting in place effective referral procedures that guarantee prompt follow-up treatment. Continuous education is also required about the appropriate use of these tests, the interpretation of findings, and the significance of confirmatory testing.

Campaigns for public health and awareness are essential in stopping the syphilis outbreak. These must be multidimensional initiatives that use a range of communication platforms and target different groups. For example, social media channels provide a chance to connect with younger demographics who could be more vulnerable. These initiatives have to concentrate on de-stigmatizing STI testing and treatment in addition to increasing public knowledge of syphilis and its symptoms.

One important aspect of these efforts is education. Many people may not be completely aware of the dangers and effects of syphilis, particularly those who are younger. Comprehensive sex education programs may provide vital knowledge about symptoms, prevention, and the value of routine testing in communities and schools. The increasing prevalence of congenital syphilis should also be addressed by these initiatives, with a focus on the value of prenatal care and testing for expectant mothers.

Reaching out specifically to groups at high risk is crucial. Working with LGBTQ+ organizations, community health facilities in underprivileged regions, and organizations that assist IV drug users are some examples of this. Messages and interventions may be more successful and reach people who are most susceptible to contracting syphilis by being tailored to certain groups.

The effect of these activities may be increased via collaborations between community groups and public health authorities. Local groups are important partners in the dissemination of knowledge and resources because they often have networks and established trust within the community. Partnerships with medical professionals, such as OB-GYNs and primary care doctors, may guarantee coordinated messaging and promote syphilis screening as a standard component of routine examinations.

One cannot stress the value of receiving expert medical follow-up. Even while at-home testing offers a preliminary screening, it cannot take the place of complete medical treatment. In order to confirm diagnoses, provide the right medication, and manage any consequences, healthcare practitioners are essential. They also provide crucial advice on partner notification and preventative techniques.

For people who test positive at home, there has to be timely access to care via simplified protocols in order to enhance the efficacy of expert follow-up. This might include expedited visits or specialized clinics for confirmation testing and therapy. Telemedicine may also be useful in facilitating early consultations and advice while scheduling follow-up appointments in person.

It is essential that healthcare personnel possess up-to-date knowledge and recommendations for the treatment of syphilis. Medical practitioners should never stop learning and growing, particularly in light of the evolving syphilis epidemiology and diagnostic techniques. This entails knowing how to interpret test findings obtained at home and knowing the proper procedures for follow-up examinations and medical intervention.

New policy ideas and developing technology will influence the future of syphilis control. The accuracy and convenience of syphilis testing are constantly being enhanced by developments in diagnostic technology. Future at-home tests may be even more dependable if research is done on more precise and sensitive testing techniques. Furthermore, advancements in point-of-care testing may provide quick, on-location confirmation testing in a variety of healthcare environments, cutting down on delays in diagnosis and treatment.

Technologies related to digital health provide encouraging paths for managing syphilis. Continued preventative efforts may be aided by mobile applications that provide information, test reminders, and connections to healthcare services. By analyzing epidemiological data, artificial intelligence and machine learning may be used to better focus treatments and anticipate epidemics.

Concerns of antibiotic resistance may be addressed as well as the effectiveness of treating syphilis by research into novel antibiotic formulations and delivery systems. For example, long-acting injectable antibiotics may enhance treatment compliance, especially in patients who may find it challenging to stick to a conventional oral antibiotic regimen.

Suggestions for policies will have a significant impact on how syphilis is controlled going forward. The need for comprehensive, national policies to combat the syphilis comeback is becoming more apparent. This involves requesting more money for research, healthcare infrastructure, and public health programs. Syphilis rates may be considerably impacted by policies that encourage broad access to testing and treatment, particularly health insurance programs that pay for at-home testing.

It is becoming more widely acknowledged that addressing the socioeconomic determinants of health is essential to the battle against syphilis. Policies that address problems like homelessness, inequality in healthcare access, and poverty may have a significant impact on STI prevalence. This all-encompassing strategy recognizes that syphilis rates often indicate more serious social and public health problems.

Another area of interest is the incorporation of syphilis screening into standard medical appointments. Guidelines for routine syphilis testing as part of yearly physicals are often included in policy recommendations, particularly for high-risk persons. Policies that encourage universal syphilis screening during prenatal care are essential for avoiding congenital syphilis in expectant mothers.

Strategies for controlling syphilis that are successful must include monitoring systems and data exchange. More timely and focused actions may result from policies that make it easier for public health organizations and hospital systems to share epidemiological data. Faster trend and epidemic hotspot identification is made possible by enhanced surveillance technologies, which facilitate prompt action.

International coordination and policy alignment are important due to the global character of the syphilis comeback. Global efforts to reduce syphilis may be strengthened by exchanging resources, research results, and best practices across national boundaries. International organizations are essential in organizing these initiatives and offering advice to nations dealing with related issues.

In the future, combating syphilis is anticipated to include a blend of technical advancement, legislative modifications, and community involvement. The persistent commitment of governments, healthcare providers, and communities is important for the success of these endeavors. Reducing syphilis rates and enhancing general sexual health must always be the top priorities as we adjust to new possibilities and challenges.

In this new environment, at-home testing is probably going to play a bigger part. These tests have the potential to drastically change how we approach STI screening and prevention as they become more accessible and broadly recognized. However, how effectively they are included into public health campaigns and comprehensive care programs will determine how successful they are.

Education and public awareness campaigns will always be essential elements of any winning plan. Our strategies for STI awareness and sexual health education must change along with societal norms and communication platforms. Keeping up the pace in the battle against syphilis may depend on engaging the younger generation via peer-led activities and internet platforms.

The continuous problem of antibiotic resistance makes the need for novel strategies to manage syphilis even more pressing. Although the efficacy of existing therapies is maintained, the possibility of resistance highlights the need for early identification and preventative tactics. The development of a vaccine and research into novel treatment options may be crucial to future attempts to reduce syphilis.

In the end, combating the syphilis recurrence will need a persistent, comprehensive strategy. Collaboration across several sectors, including public health, education, and policy, as well as healthcare, will be necessary. We can fight to reverse the trend of growing syphilis incidence and improve sexual health outcomes for everyone by using emerging technology, putting evidence-based policies into practice, and continuing to prioritize comprehensive treatment and community participation.